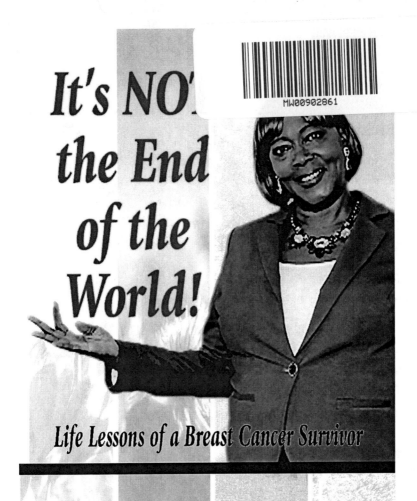

It's NOT the End of the World!

Life Lessons of a Breast Cancer Survivor

Margin Wilson

***Priority*ONE**
p u b l i c a t i o n s

Detroit, MI, USA

It's NOT the End of the World: Life Lessons of a Breast Cancer Survivor
Copyright © 2016 Margin Wilson

*Priority*ONE Publications
P. O. Box 34722 • Detroit, MI 48234
E-mail: info@priorityonebooks.com
URL: http://www.priorityonebooks.com

Hardcover
ISBN 13:   978-1-933972-51-0
ISBN 10:   1-933972-51-3

Paperback
ISBN 13:   978-1-933972-54-1
ISBN 10:   1-933972-51-8

Editing by Patricia Hicks
Cover and Interior design by Christina Dixon

Printed in the United States of America

Table of Contents

Dedication

It's May 4, 2010, I am about to start my second phase of breast cancer treatment. Two surgeries are done; chemo is about to start. I don't know what to expect, but here I go! Lord, I ask You to hold my hands.

My story is dedicated to many, but most importantly to my late mother, Katie B. Green. She died of complications from colon cancer in 2009. The book is also dedicated to my late sisters, Gail Denise Green and Linda Kay Hall. Gail died from complications of bone cancer and Linda died unexpectedly in March, 2015. I'll write more about her later in the book.

Lastly to family members still living and others. This is to my sisters, Patricia Green and Liz Richardson, and my daughter, Dionne Lenigan, as well as to women, children, and men who might be diagnosed with breast cancer or any other cancer. It is also to those who are cancer survivors. Through their stories of survival, they have inspired me to keep fighting each day that God allows me to see. Most importantly, I encourage all women to get a mammogram annually. Whether you are a man, woman, or child, please get checked by your doctor so that the cancer can be detected in its earliest stage.

Introduction

I was diagnosed with breast cancer in March of 2010 during a routine mammogram. To say the least, it was devastating news to hear. However, in some way, I knew this diagnosis of breast cancer would change my life in many ways.

I will share this cancer treatment journey with others. This was all new to me. Other than the materials I read about cancer and other survivors I had the chance to talk to on my job, along with friends, and family I didn't know what to expect.

I was devastated! I felt like screaming! Thoughts and questions started racing through my head. Oh God why me, I thought! What did I do to deserve this? How would I function? How will I survive? How will I tell my family? Will I die; is this the end for me?

However, a still soft voice whispered to me, "No Margin you will not die; this is just your season to battle breast cancer." When reading my book, you will learn about the process of my survival: my experience with two surgeries, chemotherapy, hair loss, radiation, side effects from these treatments, my hospital admissions, and my remission process.

I took comfort in God's Word which says, "To everything there is a season, a time for every purpose under the heaven... He has made everything beautiful in his time." (Ecc. 3:1-8, 11a)

Looking back, I realize that it was my season to go through breast cancer treatments. I was sick for a spell, but I got well and now I am encouraging women of the importance of getting annual mammograms.

So come walk with me as I share my walk with God down this cancer road. I will share several life lessons that I learned as I came to grips with this diagnosis. Today, I am a survivor through God's Grace!

Chapter 1

The Diagnosis

The voices and thoughts would not stop. I would constantly hear them during my quiet times. Very often, when waking up during the early morning hours, I would hear, *"You need to go get a mammogram."* Of course, I would ignore the voices. However, they would always come back to my mind. Now I know that it was the voice of God.

It wasn't until I started experiencing right shoulder pain, which would not stop, that I was prompted to make an appointment with my doctor, Dr. Peters. While there I made a mental note to be sure and ask him for an authorization to get a mammogram. I did and was immediately scheduled for an appointment in March, 2010 at my local hospital that specializes in women's health.

I promptly went one day after work. I was thinking that this would just be another annual routine mammogram, a piece of cake. Everything went smoothly, the mammogram went without incident. The films looked normal per the nurse. *"You can get dressed,"* she said. *"If there are any questions or concerns, we will call you back."* Ahhh, I thought, another mammogram over for another year!

Not so! Within a few days, I was called at work by a frantic nurse. She stated that after a second look, my mammogram showed a suspicious looking mass on the left breast. She stated that I needed to return to the center immediately. They needed to take more x-rays of the suspicious mass, and shortly after, I was scheduled for a "fine point needle biopsy." This is a process which requires a pathologist to take "tissue from a living body in order to find a diagnosis."

At this point, things started moving fast, like a roller coaster ride. The biopsy was scheduled about a week later. My anxiety level was at an all-time high; I needed time to breathe, I thought. On the day of the biopsy, I was so nervous that I was shaking. First, they had to take even more mammogram pictures to be sure the biopsy was centered at the correct site. Secondly, they walked and talked me through everything they were about to do and explained the process thoroughly. After changing into my hospital gown, I stepped up onto the hospital bed, laid sideways on the hospital bed, per direction from the nurses. Bandages and towels were placed near the area. Surrounded by nurses and pathologist, they said, "Be very still Mrs. Wilson, don't move, just a little poke, breathe and relax."

I was so afraid, and God knows I don't like needles. Just thinking of the needle sent cold chills up my spine. This was all new to me. *Lord help me*, was constantly in my mind. In that moment, God placed Psalm 46:1 on my heart, *"God is our refuge and strength, a very present help in trouble."* The nurse sensed that I was nervous, and she assured me that everything would be all right, "We will take good care of you," she said.

She was right. Once they localized the area on the left side near the mass, I felt a little pinch as the needle went in. I was numbed and felt nothing after that. I was able to relax a bit and listened to the nurses and pathologist talking in various medical terminologies that only they understood. To say the least, everything went fine!

A few days after the biopsy, I got the dreaded phone call while sitting at my desk at work.

She introduced herself as one of the nurses from the Women's Center; I braced myself for the worst. She went on to say, *"Is this Mrs. Margin Wilson?"* I said, "Yes, this is she." *"I have your reports back from the pathologist. I'm sorry Dear; it's cancer!"*

I instantly went into a state of shock, as if I was having an out-of-body experience. *She is not talking about me, Margin,* I thought; *she's got to be referring to somebody else but certainly not me! No, it can't be. No Lord!*

I was speechless! She continued, without my interruption, *"The pathologist report shows you have Invasive Ductal Carcinoma in the left breast, Stage III, and it has spread to your lymph nodes."* The nurse apologized for having to be the bearer of such bad news and informed me that I would be receiving further calls on what steps to take next. After hanging up the phone, I felt like screaming, but I couldn't; I was at work! I felt like bursting out crying, but my co-workers would think I had lost my mind. My mind was racing with thoughts of, "You are going to die." *What should I do now Lord, and why me,* I thought. What did I do to deserve this tragic news? Should I just leave work and go home? Should I tell my manager at work? Should I call my husband? I knew if I did any of the above at that point, I was going to burst out crying uncontrollably. I definitely was going to lose it!

For the next few hours after that call, I tried to pretend to be working. I tried not to let the tears fall in front of my coworkers. I tried to smile and be calm and happy, like everything was okay, just another Monday morning at work. Everything I attempted to do brought tears to my eyes. My heart was so heavy to the point of aching, and I couldn't keep it in any longer. My manager, Mary, approached me and asked me how was I doing. I tearfully and emotionally explained to her about the call I received earlier, and I could feel the tears starting to roll profusely down my cheeks. I began to cry like a baby, uncontrollably on Mary's shoulders. I didn't care anymore about being at work or who heard or saw me crying. At that point, I just needed a shoulder to cry on. She hugged me, telling me she was so sorry to hear that I had cancer, and that everything would be okay. Other coworkers began to come and comfort me at that moment as well as give me encouraging words.

Mary even confided in me that she had been diagnosed with cancer a few years before. She stated I was going to be fine. She reiterated that when I was ready to talk about it, she could give me some knowledge on what she went through with her treatments. She also mentioned other coworkers at work who had dealt with cancer or had a family member who had cancer and that I could get good advice from them also. God was already working and sending people to my rescue. God steps right in when you need

Him; "He may not come when you want Him, but He's right on time.[1]"

I immediately told my husband, family, and friends after leaving work that day. My husband also reassured me that we were going to go through this together, no matter what. My children were very supportive, as well as my brothers, sisters, and other family members. Family sent out prayers, and I got words of encouragement from friends almost immediately. God is so good, I thought! He will send you help that you don't know about from all directions.

---

[1] The Best of Dorothy Love Coates & The Original Gospel Harmonettes, *You Can't Hurry God,* 2006

Notes

Chapter 2

Preparing for Surgery

So now I have to schedule an appointment with my doctor, Dr. Peters, so he can refer me to an authorized surgeon. In the process of meeting with my doctor, I had to schedule time off work, fill out medical papers for work, and make sure my diabetes was under control. I was told my surgery would be cancelled if my blood sugar or blood pressure were too high. I needed my shots up to date. I had a flu shot, pneumonia shot, tetanus shot, insulin shot, and an EKG done.

After all these procedures were completed, my surgeon, Dr. Ethan, was introduced to me. He was a very good, well qualified cancer surgeon, from what I was told by Dr. Peters. In April of 2010, an appointment was scheduled, and I met with him at the Josephine Ford Cancer Center, located in West Bloomfield Hills, Michigan. Dr. Ethan appeared to be very concerned about my condition and tried to reassure me that everything would be all right.

As he introduced himself to me, we shook hands and courteously smiled at each other; and he began to explain exactly what my diagnosis entailed. After sitting down at his desk, he immediately pulled out a green booklet, which talked about breast cancer. He began by saying, *"Mrs. Wilson, you have what is called, Invasive Ductal Carcinoma of the left breast and it has spread to your lymph nodes."* He opened up the green booklet and there was a picture of a woman's breast, shoulder, and arm. He began to mark the areas on the breast where the surgeries would take place and where approximately the cancer was located. Three surgeries would be performed. He reiterated that it was on the left side, drawing a mark in the center of the breast.

The first surgery we would remove the actual cancer in the left breast. Then he drew a mark underneath the upper left armpit. The second surgery was called an Axillary Node Surgery, where the lymph nodes would be removed. This involved a slight incision underneath the left armpit. Nodes were removed to see how far the cancer had spread. The third surgery involved the insertion of a Power Port inside the right chest area to prepare me for chemotherapy. He explained that a port is an object that is inserted underneath the skin, in order to insert the IV needle for chemotherapy. Dr. Ethan asked me if I had any questions. I took out my list!

I had a few questions of my own for Dr. Ethan:

"When is my surgery?"

"Your surgery is scheduled for April 22, 2010."

"Where will the surgery take place?"

"Here, at Henry Ford Hospital, West Bloomfield, Michigan."

"What stage is my cancer?"

"Your cancer is around Stage II which is an early stage."

"Will I have to be put to sleep?"

"General Surgery under local anesthesia. Yes, you will be put to sleep."

"Will I have an overnight stay or outpatient surgery?"

"This will be an outpatient procedure."

As we ended our question and answer period, Dr. Ethan smiled and said, "Don't forget to sign the green book. It's yours. It has good information inside for you to read about breast cancer and what to expect."

Notes

Chapter 3

Day of Surgery

It's 6:30 a.m. Thursday morning, April 22, 2010, still dark outside, a very cool April morning, and the day of my surgery. Walter, my husband, and Dionne, my daughter, were riding with me to the hospital. Once we arrived, we checked in at the Information Desk. We were then greeted by a hospital staff person who escorted us to the elevator that would take us up to the Surgery Department. In route, he began to give us a brief tour of the newly built Food Court located on the first floor of the hospital.

I felt really nervous at this point. I didn't know what to expect at this moment. Would the surgery go well? How long would I be under anesthesia? What would I see when the elevator doors opened up to the Second Floor Surgery Department? My heart was pumping and thumping really fast! God help me, went through my mind repeatedly!

The elevator door opened! There was a sea of nurses, doctors, and patients surrounding various cubicles with hospital beds throughout the room. There were two or three nurses sitting at the patient's desk laughing, talking, and discussing patient information. I looked around at the patients waiting for their surgeries. They were already dressed from head to toe in their hospital garb: cap, gown, shoes, IV bag, and surrounded by their own family members. The greeter who rode up with us on the elevator introduced me to a nurse, "She will be taking care of you from this point on," he said.

"My name is Carol," she said, as she began to walk me to my designated cubicle. She gave me a bag to put my clothes in. Also, she gave me the hospital garb: cap, gown, and shoes. She pointed me to the bathroom where I changed my clothes. As I walked towards the bathroom, I could really start to feel my heart racing. I was feeling a lot of anxiety at this point. I know there's no turning back; I was afraid and nervous! After changing my clothes, I headed back to my cubicle where my husband and daughter were waiting.

A different nurse then came in and greeted us with a "Good Morning!" She introduced herself and proceeded to take my blood pressure, checked my blood sugar, and put the IV in my arm. After about an hour, other nurses came in to check on me and to give me instructions on what would shortly be taking place. The Anesthesiologist came in and took a seat; she had many questions, instructions, and ran me through General Anesthesia procedures and precautions. I knew the time for surgery was drawing near and felt good that things would be over shortly.

My surgeon, Dr. Ethan, finally arrived. Pulling the cubicle curtains back, he appeared, like the invisible man, standing in front of me with a slight smile on his face. He reassured me that all would go well, my surgery was up next, and for me not be nervous. "Everything will be all right. I will take good care of you. Don't be nervous," he said. Putting on his surgical cap, he walked toward the surgery room. The sea of nurses surrounded my hospital bed and I said goodbye to my husband and daughter. They prepared me to go in for surgery, no turning back, and once again I thought, *Lord Help Me!*

Lights are everywhere inside the surgical room. Nurses and doctors surrounded my hospital bed. In unison, counting 1,2,3, they slid me onto the table. I could hear pop music playing in the background, along with the doctors and nurses talking and laughing among themselves. Both my arms were stretched out across the surgical table. The anesthesiologist said to me, "We are going to put you to sleep for a little while; just relax."

Dr. Ethan asked me what type of music I wanted to hear before I went to sleep. "We have R&B, Pop, Country, Motown, whatever you want to hear," he said. I said, "Jesus Take the Wheel" by Carrie Underwood. As I began to fall asleep I heard "Jesus Take the Wheel" playing in the background. I could feel the hands of one of the nurses rubbing the side of my cheeks, she said, "Go to sleep; we will take good care of you."

Notes

Chapter 4

After Surgery

I felt really good after surgery. I stayed in Recovery a couple of hours. I was all bandaged up around my chest and arms where the surgery was done, but I felt no pain, just a little wobbly and dizzy. Everything went well, however, I was so sleepy that I didn't want to move. I could hear the nurse telling me, "Wake up Mrs. Wilson, wake up! You have to get up and get dressed." Once I finally opened my eyes I could see my husband and daughter sitting next to me. They were also trying to get me to wake up. I think I told the nurse that the doctor had said I could stay overnight. She quickly informed me this was an outpatient procedure and I needed to wake up, get dressed, and prepare to go home!

About three weeks after recovering at home from the surgery, I returned to Dr. Ethan's office for my 3-week checkup. He told me that he had some good news and some bad news. The good news was that the surgery went fine. The bad news was that the pathologist report showed there was about a centimeter of the cancer that was missed. They would have to do a second surgery, which is called a re-excision, to remove the rest of the cancer. I could feel the tears starting to well up in my eyes, and my doctor handed me the box of tissues. I could not believe I had to go through surgery again. I was in a state of shock at that moment! God help me, I thought! Dr. Ethan reassured me that in some cases this does happen and routinely a second surgery is immediately scheduled.

The second surgery was scheduled about two weeks later. The same routine was followed as the first surgery. Only this time, things seemed to go faster. Seemingly, the surgery was over in a matter of minutes. During Recovery, I could hear the nurse saying, "Wake up Mrs. Wilson, it's time to get dressed." In my groggy state, I managed to get up out of the bed, put on my clothes by myself, and once she pulled the curtain back, she was startled to see me dressed and ready to go. Yes, God brought me through, once again, safe and sound!

My Season, My Thoughts

Thus far, God has brought me through four surgeries. He blessed me so that everything has gone well. All the cancer has been removed. I can say right now; I am cancer free! Lymph nodes were removed and a drain tube inserted under my left arm. A lumpectomy was performed so that only the cancer was removed and not the whole breast, thank God!

Also, I had a Power Port inserted surgically underneath the skin on my right chest for use once chemotherapy began. My family and friends were praying for me constantly. I received cards, flowers, fruit baskets and well wishes from family, friends, and co-workers.

Most of all, I know God is still holding my hand as I journey down this road. Thank you Jesus!

Chapter 5

Chemotherapy

I learned my oncologist would be a Dr. Adams. Before actually meeting Dr. Adams, I had to see several Oncology Specialists, two to be exact. Their job was to give me the ins and outs of what chemotherapy would entail. Their synopsis was for me to imagine beautiful green grass being invaded by yellow dandelions. See the dandelions as various cells in your body. We don't know which cell has been affected by the cancer, since the cancer had spread to the lymph nodes. Therefore, we have to spray weed killer on all those cells, which would be the chemotherapy drugs. In the process of killing the bad cells, some good cells may be affected in the process.

After seeing the specialists, I had my first appointment with Dr. Adams. He explained the various chemo drugs he would be using for my treatment. Again, I was warned about the side effects. I was greeted by one of the RN Nurses, Martha. She also gave me an informal prep-meeting about the chemo treatments I would be receiving there at the clinic. She provided me with various books, pamphlets, and brochures on what to expect during the seven treatments. I saw a brief video of previous cancer patients explaining their experiences during chemo treatment.

They talked about the hair loss, weight loss, nausea, vomiting, and loss of appetite. They explained that all of the above occurs in the process of the chemo trying to kill off those bad cells. Was I prepared for all of this? No, I was not!

My first chemo treatment started at 10:00 a.m. on June 18, 2010. I was feeling a little anxious and a little nervous at the same time. Of course, I was expecting the worst but was attempting to stay upbeat! It was a nice, sunshiny beautiful day. My husband, Walter, and daughter, Dionne were with me. I had not eaten any breakfast fearing I would be late for this first appointment.

Once arriving inside the clinic, I checked in with the receptionist. She handed me an I.D. badge to put on my arm, I took a seat, and waited for my name to be called. In the process of waiting, my daughter went and got me some breakfast. I was informed that the treatment would be between two to three hours long. I heard my name called, looked around, and was greeted by a nurse who expressed a very inviting smile.

Walking behind her, we entered a back spacious room with lots of windows. She asked me if I would like a private room or sit out in this spacious area with lots of windows. Of course, I chose the private room.

Everything appeared to be running smoothly. I was still feeling good. I had my husband and daughter with me, and I even had my own private room. The room displayed a big picture glass window that looked out onto a beautiful flower patio garden. Equipped with a running fountain, there were little birds flying under the fountain to bath themselves. There were colorful flowers of yellow, orange, and pink situated around the garden. For a moment, the look and feel of my surroundings outside my window, took my mind off of what I was about to encounter.

The nurse walked in as I reared back onto the lazy boy recliner. She explained to me the types of chemo drugs that would be administered. She first had to flush out the power port using that awful smelling saline solution, which always made me nauseous. "I hope you had breakfast," she said. I implied my daughter had left to get me breakfast. The nurse proceeded to inform me of the three drugs. One IV bag was a reddish color and two bags were a clear liquid.

She also informed me that my treatment would last about three hours. She proceeded to hand me a warm blanket and pillow. I was loving the attention, but dreaded the inevitable.

Feeling for my power port by pressing down on the right side of my chest, the nurse found it and began flushing it out. After flushing out the port, she drew blood from it which was immediately sent to the lab. Looking at my blood filling up the syringe I thought to myself, the power port is working just fine.

The nurse then hung the three bags of chemo drugs onto the IV Machine. First, she set the clear bags to be administered. The bag of red chemo drugs would be administered last. At this point, my daughter walked in with my breakfast. *So far, so good*, I thought. Everything was running smoothly, and at this point I felt just fine! Little did I know, drama was about to hit!

Before the drama started, I must say my first day of chemo was going better than I expected.

The three hours were going by pretty fast. I relaxed in the reclining chair and watched TV, talking and laughing with my husband and daughter. Being with my family took my mind off of the chemo drugs going into my system.

By the time I was done, I was still feeling pretty good. I felt the same as when I came in that morning. I felt no dizziness and no weakness. If anything, I was hungry again being that it was way past lunchtime. The only disappointing news was the nurse informing me that I would have to come in the next day to get a Neupogen injection, and the next four days after that.

So there I was, trying to understand what the nurse had just told me about coming in for the next five days to get a shot. The injection, the nurse explains is to keep my blood platelets high, so the levels won't get too low during chemotherapy treatments.

By the afternoon, my first chemo was over and done. The sun was still shining bright as ever. I still felt normal, and I was really hungry! We stopped at a local store to get some items the nurse said I might need. I purchased a Vernor's soda pop (just in case I experienced any nausea), a thermometer (just in case a fever occurred), and a large bag of potato chips (just for a late snack). I was thinking all the while this chemo "is just a piece of cake."

We stopped at a local eatery to get lunch. I wanted a chicken salad sandwich, along with a bowl of clam chowder, and a medium diet pop. My husband and I shared lunch on the back deck of our home. I was still enjoying the day and just feeling fine, telling myself that my first chemo was now history!

Notes

Chapter 6

Chemo Aftermath

Closer to the evening, I ate dinner and went to bed. Around 3 a.m., I was awakened with a severe case of nausea. My hand reached over to the waste basket pulling it closer to me and the bed. I could feel everything I had eaten the day before about to expel themselves. Here it comes, I thought!

All I could do was bury my head inside the basket and, "let her go." It was coming none stop. As soon as I thought it was done, the vomiting would start up again. Yes, the chemo drugs seemed to be attacking everything I had congested. When my mind would think about any food, I would vomit.

For about five to ten minutes, I was really, really sick! I began to get weaker and dehydrated. The chemo made it impossible for me to even keep water down. When I would drink water, that too, came up.

My husband soon said, "get dressed, we are going to Emergency." It was 4 a.m. in the morning. I was still feeling nauseated, so I took a vomit bag alone with me while riding in the car. Once arriving to Emergency, I checked in at the front desk. Shortly after, I was called to the back room by the nurse.

As the nurse began to ask me what brought me there, I attempted to answer, and started vomiting once again. Thank

God, I had that vomit bag with me. Still feeling very sick, the nurse put me in an empty room with a bed to lie down. No sooner I laid down, I was up vomiting again. A different nurse then entered my room and said she would get me something to stop the nausea.

She brought me a tablet and told me to place it under my tongue and let it dissolve. I tried to explain to her, it's not going to work because my stomach could not stand anything. Once the minty tasting of the tablet hit the bottom of my stomach, it starts up again. I was now feeling miserable! As if that wasn't enough, the nurse said I have something else I want you to try, of course, that didn't work either.

After being in Emergency for a couple of hours, the nurse and staff started up the regular routine. They took blood work, IV hook up, blood pressure, taking my temperature, etc. I was trying to get some rest and get comfortable. Shortly after, the nurse entered stating the doctor is going to admit you to the hospital.

I was thinking in my mind; *this must be serious.* The nurses began to prep me for Admission. I was going to be transported, by Ambulance, to the major hospital downtown. No sooner the prepping was done, I looked up and two tall male transporters, dressed in identical white and black uniforms, are walking towards my bed. They too, also have their transporter's bed that they roll in with them. They hand me a bag for my belongings, asking me if I have everything.

Making sure I was comfortable, they switched me from the hospital's bed to their transporter's bed. They told me to take my time and just slide over. Then they proceeded to buckle me in, stating this is procedure to make sure you don't fall out once we lift you up into the transporter's van.

What's next, I thought! Once inside the Ambulance, EMS workers check my blood pressure, check my blood sugar, again. They assure me everything will be alright, and just to relax, I did!

My Season, My Thoughts

My first bout with chemotherapy was rough, to say the least, but God was still with me.

It made me realize that sometimes when you are not in that position to pray for yourself, prayers have already gone up on my behalf.

Prayers my Mom prayed, prayers I prayed, prayers my Pastor prayed, preachers, mothers of the church, missionaries of the church, and many others have laid prayers up on my behalf, "for such a time as this."

My mother used to always say to me, "I anoint myself and pray for my children every day." I say, "Thank You God for storing up my mother's prayers on my behalf. I have a Spiritual Bank Account and now I have to withdraw from it. A lot have been deposited. I need it right now!"

Notes

Chapter 7
In the Hospital, First Time

After being admitted into the hospital, the nurse began to hook me up to the IV monitor machine. She told me her name, Robin, and that she was going to be my nurse for the rest of the day shift. She handed me a hospital gown, slippers, and toiletries needed for my stay. She introduced me to her nursing assistant, Sheila, who proceeded to give me extra gowns and blankets that I might need.

Robin began looking at my medical chart and mentioned the fact that I had been experiencing non-stop vomiting. She stated that she would have to my talk with my doctor, who would prescribe something to stop the vomiting. Sheila checked my blood pressure, blood sugar, and stated that I would need to urinate inside the white pail located in the bathroom; which she would need to check every day. Before she left, I asked her for ice water.

After not being able to keep anything on my stomach, I became very dehydrated and thirsty; and not for just cold water either. It had to have ice in it. That's all my system wanted at that point.

Later that afternoon, Robin puts medicine in my IV to help with my nausea. Before that process, my power port (which is connected to the IV) has to be flushed out with Saline Solution.

However, the smell of saline upsets my stomach once again. In trying to block out the smell with a wash cloth, I still caught a swift of it and started vomiting again. Robin rushed to get me a pail and apologized.

By the next morning, around 8 a.m., I awoke to a team of doctors coming towards my bed wearing white coats. Dr. Howard, the head doctor, asked me how I was feeling. I told him I was feeling better. He explains that he hoped the medicine he prescribed was working. I replied that it was working. He replies, "We are going to take care of you." He reassures me if I needed anything or have any questions, just let the nurses know. Once the vomiting is under control, that I would be released but I would have to try and eat something.

Dr. Howard explains that it is very important to try and eat something. That they needed to know the food is staying down and that the medication was working. I told him I would try. However, I could not stand the smell of any food. I could smell eggs and bacon that morning and I was about to vomit. A tray of eggs, bacon, tea and toast were brought to my bedside, and I quickly pushed it away. I did eventually drink the hot tea, however, when lunch and dinner came around it was hot tea again and of course, my ice water.

On the second morning, I felt a little better than the day before. Once again, I couldn't eat the breakfast. For lunch, I thought I would try a liquid soup. To my surprise the soup stayed down. Dinner was mash potatoes and beef which was a struggle to stay down but stayed down none the less. I felt the medication was finally working!

On the third day, I was up walking up and down the hallway floors near my room. I was feeling less weak and feeling more energetic. Other patients were also up and walking the floors. I felt so much better. The vomiting had subsided somewhat and I could be discharged by noon. I even felt my appetite coming back and requested vegetable soup for lunch.

During the process of packing up for discharge my lunch arrived. I hurried and ate my lunch and really felt better. About 30 minutes later, all the soup came up! I figured I was eating too fast. Once at home, I have to focus on taking things very slow when eating solid foods.

Notes

Chapter 8

Home Again!

Once home, I remembered that right after chemo treatment, there's two weeks of feeling really crappy and weak. This includes, vomiting, diarrhea, loss of appetite, dizziness, weakness, and all you want to do is stay in bed and be left alone. On the other hand, there's two weeks of feeling normal. This includes feeling energetic, good appetite, wanting to get up and move about, not dizzy, and just feeling strength in your body, alert and alive.

At this point, your body is going through so many changes. As if feeling nauseated wasn't enough, I had to force myself to eat. I would go a whole day without eating and without being hungry. I knew I had to try and eat something. Amazingly, when I did manage to eat a little something, my food didn't taste the same. I remembered trying to eat a hot dog, it was tasteless! It reminded me of having a bad cold and you lose your sense of smell. You can't smell or taste anything.

I know how meatloaf taste, a bag of potato chips, a bowl of corn flakes, etc. However, nothing I was eating tasted right. At least for the first two weeks right after chemo, all my food was tasteless. The only thing that tasted the same was water. I could not get enough of ice water. However, in order for my body to get stronger, I knew I had to eat. As I began to eat, I could feel my body strength returning.

In fact, whereas I couldn't bath myself without being tired and out of breath, now I could see that this was subsiding. I didn't have to actually take a break and sit down in the middle of bathing or washing up. After brushing my teeth, the taste of toothpaste would cause my stomach to be upset, that eventually stopped. As my body regained its strength from eating, I felt so much better. Even swallowing my diabetic pills in the morning stayed down and I didn't vomit them up.

My daily routine, after chemo, caused me to take things very slowly. Although strength was returning, going up and down stairs was challenging. I just took my time, taking one step at a time. I knew everything was a little different now with my eating, washing, bathing, just trying to feel normal again. I Thank God for giving me the strength to make it this far!

I could feel my appetite returning. I could feel certain food taste coming back to normal. Boy, it was good to taste meatloaf again! I could eat without vomiting. The nausea was subsiding and my stomach didn't feel upset. I felt like getting up in the morning. I was motivated to do something. Just having the feeling of wanting and feeling like doing something was good enough for me.

I got up and dressed myself. I did laundry. I washed dishes. I swept the kitchen floor and mopped as well. I fixed dinner and was able to eat it, with taste buds intact. I could go up and down the stairs, catching my breath on occasions, but I kept going. I was just so thankful I was up and moving about.

Home Again!

I learned with chemo, you have to fight for your strength. You have to fight to live and be normal again. If you let it, chemo can consume you. Rest when you need to. It's a must that you eat, because your appetite will leave you for a while. Drink plenty of water. And by all means, keep moving!!!!!

My Season, My Thoughts

God was on my side as I went through chemotherapy treatments. I was hospitalized for a spell, but God brought me out. Sometimes I would feel all alone, but God would always reassure me that He was with me all the way.

My husband, Walter, and family were a blessing too. My husband stayed by my bedside in the hospital. My kids came to help with my needs at home. My brothers and sisters would come by the house or call to check on me. Friends would call or send "Get Well" cards. Thank God for family and friends!

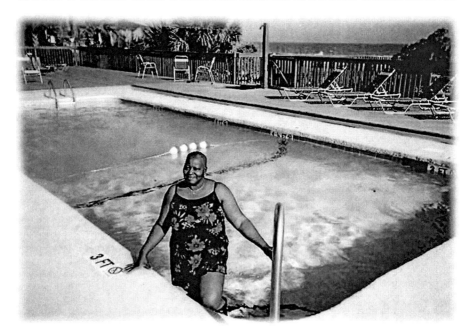

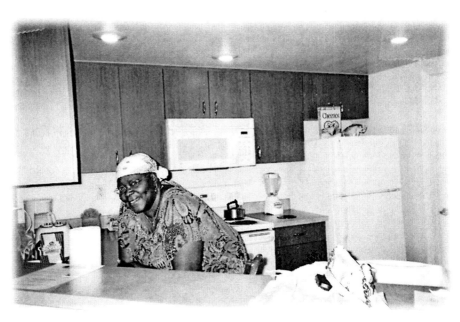

Chapter 9

Hair Loss

It was around July 2, 2010, that my hair started falling out. I would comb my hair and big chunks of hair would come out in the sink. I stopped combing and brushing my hair for fear of what I would see. Little by little, I would see hair just falling out, even when I didn't comb or brush it. It got so bad, all I had to do was pull my hair and it would just come out. It was sort of like cotton candy when you pull on it to eat it. That's what my hair felt like.

Of course, I was devastated! No hair! *What would people think*, I thought! How would I feel when I became completely bald? I felt so sad, so torn inside. But what could I do but go on and hold my head up high.

I would pin what little hair I had left, up with bobby pins. I wore a baseball cap on some days. The only hair left was my front bang, which I just pushed to the front to show I had a little hair left. I was desperately trying to hold on to what little hair I had left as long as I could. Eventually, I had to face the inevitable.

One morning, I woke up and just started pulling out the remaining hair. In a matter of minutes, all the hair I could pull out was gone. Some remaining patchy spots of hair were left but I was unable to pull them out. The next step was to make an appointment with my beautician, Gladys.

I was told up front that chemo would eventually take my hair out, but when it actually happens, it's an unbelievable, surreal feeling. All I could do was ask God for strength to endure. I had purchased some colorful scarfs of red, pink, green, black, and white along with a wig. I think physically I had prepared for the hair loss but mentally it was going to be an experience that I just had to go through. The shame, embarrassment, low self-esteem, and insecurities hit me all at once.

I had to do like David in 1 Samuel 30:6, "encourage myself in the Lord." I'm beautiful, anyhow! Psalm 118:6 says, "God is on my side." And our Father has told us in Hebrews 13:5, "I will never leave you or forsake you." I figured I would just have to reinvent myself for the better. To help me do that, I finally made that appointment with Gladys.

I told Gladys that all my hair had fallen out from chemotherapy treatments. After taking my scarf off to show her, she said, "That is alright you're still beautiful. We are going to fix you up." She then proceeded to get the clippers and shaved the rest of the patchy spots of hair off. It didn't take long, only a few minutes. As she placed my scarf back on my head and tied it in one of her stylish fashions, she reassured me as she whispered that everything would be alright. I shook my head in agreement with her and walked out of her shop feeling really encouraged!

I must say, there are some positives about being bald. First, I saved $90 not having to get my hair done. Secondly, I didn't have to worry about rolling my hair or using the hot curlers daily. Thirdly, I could actually have the window down and not worry about the wind messing my hair up. It felt so good to ride in the front seat of the car and just let the wind blow, blow, blow! Furthermore, when my scalp itched, there was easy access for scratching. Also, washing the scalp was a breeze; no blow drying!

The next few months during that summer, I noticed the hair on my body was disappearing. I lost my eyebrows. I lost my eyelashes. All facial hair was gone. I didn't have to shave armpits or legs. Without a doubt, I can say wherever hair grew on my body, the chemotherapy took it all away. In the midst of it all, God gave me strength!

To this day, all of my hair has come back, except my eyebrows. I had really dark, soft eyebrows, which I really miss to this day. Some things we take for granted, and when they are gone, we really regret it. One thing I learned when I lost my eyelashes was that they help to control the tear ducts in the eye. My eyes would always tear up before the eyelashes grew back. I asked the nurse during one office visit and she gave that information to me. I was so glad to know it, because I thought I was going blind during the day when the sun was bright.

I carried tissue constantly to wipe my eyes. At times things would appear blurry. I would blink a lot trying to see clearly. In the morning when I woke up, I felt I was in a daze because I wasn't seeing clearly. It was a scary time for me. However, it all went back to normal once my eyelashes grew back.

Notes

Chapter 10

Back in the Hospital

The nurse reiterated to me, "You know after each of your chemo treatments, you have to come in for the next five days to get your Neupogen injections. I replied, "No," because I didn't know. "Your doctor should have told you that." She began to schedule me for the next five days which, mind you, included Saturday and Sunday.

I was devastated to say the least! However, of course, I gathered up enough strength to go in and get my injections. I was feeling nauseated from the chemo. However, I went in five days in a row and got this stinky, irritating injection in the back of my arm. Did I mention, that I absolutely hate needles and shots?

After getting my last of the five injections and while at home, I began experiencing muscle pain. It started in my neck and moved down my back. I attempted to rest a bit, thinking the pain would go away. But it would not go away. I called Emergency because the pain was becoming unbearable. I was told by the on-call doctor that the muscle pain was one of the side effects from the Neupogen injections. Within a couple of days, the pain should subside. It didn't!

On Sunday of the following week, a friend and spiritual evangelist of the family, Marcie, prayed with me that the pain would go away, in Jesus' Name! Before me and my husband left for dinner that night, the muscle pain had completely left. The pain did not return, thank God!

After that, I was back in the hospital for the second time. With the chemo treatments, I could not keep my food down. This was still going on after my third chemo treatment. Once again, I ended up in Emergency and stayed practically throughout the night trying to get the vomiting under control. Finally, the nurse said, "The doctor is going to admit you."

I was transported by EMS to the Main Hospital downtown. I went through the same procedure as before. Once arriving at the Main Hospital, I was rolled onto the stretcher, rolled down the long hallways to my room, and given a hospital gown to change into. My blood pressure was checked, sugar checked, and now the paperwork began. While all of this was going on, I felt another episode of vomiting was about to explode! All I wanted was a nice, cold glass of ice water. I was so thirsty and dehydrated.

After three days in the hospital, my appetite started to return. The nurses had been trying to get me to eat something, but I was so nauseated that food was the last thing I wanted. Meanwhile, gradually I could feel my appetite coming back. I started with a cup of tea, a bowl of cereal, and for lunch a cup of broth. I was so glad that all the food stayed down. I was happy that the medicines they had put in my IV were finally working. I started to feel normal again!

I was kept in the hospital a little longer this time. It was four days. I assumed the doctors really wanted to be sure my stomach had settled and the vomiting stopped before they discharged me. The nurses were constantly putting various medicines in my IV to make sure I felt better.

I was so proud that my husband stayed by my side, all the while I was in the hospital. After working his 8 hours, and sometimes overtime, he would come to the hospital and spend the night with me in my room. The hospital supplied a recliner that also facilitated as a bed. This was so comforting to me.

On the day of my discharge, patiently waiting for all my prescriptions to be cleared (it took a long time for my medicines to come up to my room), I later learned that there was some type of discrepancy going on. Once everything cleared, I was wheeled outside to 100-degree weather. The nurse wheeling me out asked, "Is there anything I can get you?" I said yes, "Ice water."

Notes

Chapter 11

Chemo Is Done!

All together I had seven treatments of chemotherapy. They started in June of 2010 and ended in September of the same year. Each and every time I went for treatments, I got sick. I remember the nausea would be the first side effect, then weakness the second culprit, and loss of appetite would be the third.

I so dreaded going to chemotherapy. Why? For the various reasons listed above, along with the fact that I would literally be bed bound for the first two weeks right after chemo. I was constantly craving ice water. At that point, I couldn't taste my food, so why even try to eat, I would think in my mind. I was irritable and didn't wish to talk to anyone because of the way I was feeling. I was really trying to sleep away the pain, which I now know, was the wrong thing to do.

There were three methods used to treat my breast cancer: Surgery; Chemotherapy; and Radiation. The most difficult treatment was the chemotherapy. During this treatment, I lost all my hair. When I say ALL my hair, that means everywhere. My fingernails turned black. My energy level went down, body was weak, dizzy spells, and I was winded when moving around. Just two weeks of being miserable.

As I gradually regained my strength, I still didn't feel quite normal. My energy level was low, felt dizzy, sluggish, and weak. To my surprise, as I began to feel normal, it was time for chemo again. I had to stop by the Lab to make sure my platelets didn't get too low.

So when I say chemo was done, it covers a lot of physical, emotional, and mental pains that come with the treatments.

On the very last day of my chemo treatment, I was so overjoyed! The nurses were overjoyed as well, along with the nurses and staff in the Oncology Department. As I walked in for the last treatment, it was announced by the nursing staff, "This is Margin Wilson's last day of chemo," one of the nurses chanted. I walked in the room to a faint applause by other patients hooked up to their IV's. I was happy to know it was just about over. I did my last treatment with ease of mind and relief. I felt so relieved that I could start living again. "Thank you Lord," I said, "Thank you Lord!"

My Season, My Thoughts

Well Lord, I say Thank You. Thank You for bringing me this far through this cancer journey! Some days I felt I wasn't going to make it through, but You brought me out! I came "this far by faith, leaning on the Lord.[2]"

I was at the point where I couldn't take being in the Chemo Lab. The smells of medicines, the sound of the IV machines pumping

---

[2] © 1965 Albert A. Goodman, *We've Come This Far by Faith*

chemo in the body, saline solution used to clean my port, which made me sick of the stomach every time I smelled it, and looking at other cancer patients hooked up to those machines just made my skin crawl!

What irritated me the most was the clicking sound of those IV machines. Also, when one patient's bag of chemo ran out, then the machine would beep until the nurse came to stop it. My chemo treatment consisted of three bags of drugs, so I sat for about three hours for each treatment. So for the change of each bag, I heard a lot of clicking and beeping. In fact, even now I cringe when I think of those moments, sitting in that recliner chair waiting for those three hours to end. However, I'm here to say, Thank God I made it!

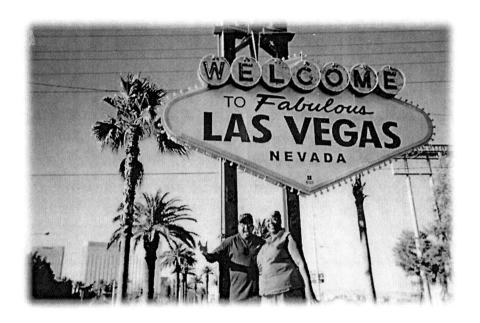

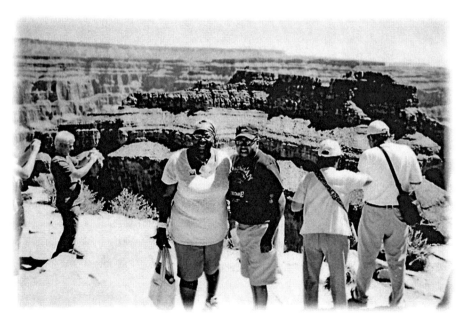

Chapter 12

A Time to Rest

In August of 2010, in the midst of my third chemo treatment, I was in bed trying to regain my strength. My husband called me on the phone. "Guess what honey," he happily said on the other end of the phone. In my mind I was thinking, *what is he up to now?*

I anxiously but momentarily came out of my feeling sick state and say, "What honey?" He then continued without hesitation and with even more enthusiasm, "We are going to Vegas," he said with great excitement. *You have got to be kidding,* I thought in my mind! He stated, "I got the plane tickets, resort rooms, and we are all set to go for seven days."

In my mind, I felt excited about being able to get away from the hospital, doctors, sick people, being in bed all day, weakness, nausea, and just the whole gamut of things I had been going through. On the other hand, I thought, *how in the world am I going to be able to make it in Vegas as sick as I was* feeling at the time.

The thought of the up and coming get-a-way gave me a boost of energy that I didn't expect. I was determined to start feeling better really fast. With all the strength I could muster up, I began to feel better each day. I fought through the weakness and fought through the feelings of being so tired. I got up and started moving! I was determined, through the Grace of God to get better, slowly but surely.

I started washing clothes, gathering our suit cases, and packing for my husband and for myself. I even did a little shopping for some of things we needed for the trip. The Las Vegas trip was on! We made it to Vegas safely and had a great time. I am so thankful that the trip was during the week chemo was not required and most of my strength and a feeling of normalcy had returned.

It was a wonderful feeling to eat and be able to actually taste my food while in Vegas. We went shopping, sightseeing at the Grand Canyon, played the slot machines, and saw a couple of shows, one in particular was Cirque du Soleil. We did some walking in 119-degree weather. The trip took my mind off of being sick, and God really blessed!

To add to that, in October of that same year, about a month after my last chemo, I got another unexpected call from my husband.

"Guess where we are going for our 30th wedding anniversary?"

"Where?" I asked.

"Myrtle Beach," he said with excitement once again.

I had never been to Myrtle Beach but had heard so much about it. I was so happy my chemo was over with at this point and really looked forward to going on another trip.

God blessed again and gave me the strength I needed to pack, wash clothes, shop for trip items, and eventually we were well on our way once again. It just let me know, in the midst of your sickness, God can come in with an unexpected blessing.

Notes

Chapter 13

Radiation

My last form of treatment for breast cancer was radiation. This was in late November of 2010, around the Thanksgiving Holiday. Radiation would require seven (7) straight weeks, starting at 11:30 a.m. for about an hour each day, except weekends and holidays. This treatment would go on throughout the Christmas Season and past New Year's.

Around this time, I met with Dr. Larry at Josephine Ford Treatment Center in West Bloomfield Hills, Michigan. He explained to me the procedure and what all it entailed. He performed a formal breast exam of my surgical scar, updated my medical history, and introduced me to the nurse who would give me further instructions.

I was introduced to the other medical staff and assistants who would be handling my radiation treatments. First, they would have to insert small needles surrounding the area where the radiation would be done. Of course, this did not sit well with me! I thought to myself, *here we go again with these needles.* However, the nurses assured me that once they marked the areas, this procedure would be a one-time deal.

The next seven (7) weeks would be "a piece of cake." So I did squirm and scream until all the needles were marked and placed. After that, I had a sigh of relief until my next appointment.

Once started, radiation required me checking in on time, head to the Locker Room to put on a hospital gown, and take a seat in the waiting area until my name was called. Everything happened like clockwork. I felt like I was on an assembly line, then I heard my name being called. "Mrs. Wilson you're next."

A soft-spoken nurse politely asked, "How are you doing? Come right in," she said. We talked for a bit and then radiation began. I took one step up onto the radiation bed, which was a flat, narrow bed covered with white sheets. The Radiation Room was equipped with different types of electronic, circular machinery. The narrow bed was surrounded by a big, white, round-shaped x-ray machine.

As I lay on the bed, very still, the x-ray machine would move, circling around my body. Up and around my head and chest, taking pictures as it circled around. The areas where the needles had been marked, it seemingly knew where to go. At various points the machine would stop, and I noticed the white laser light shining directly down on my chest. The white shining dot reminded me of a laser gun.

The nurse insisted I be very still. When I was told to be still, my body wanted to move. My nose begins to itch or my back would cramp up due to lying down in one spot for a long time. However, I felt no pain, just a little warmth from the glare of the laser lights.

Radiation

Radiation continued on for the seven weeks. Eventually, the skin on the left side of my chest, neck, and shoulder began to burn. However, I was told this could possibly happen as time went on, so I wasn't too surprised. The burns did itch terribly, peeled, and became very irritated for a couple of weeks.

The nurses informed me on how to keep the areas clean. They gave me soothing ointment to apply to the areas. Eventually, all the areas healed and cleared up. Radiation was over, thank God!

My Season, My Thoughts

At this point, I was getting close to the end of these treatments. Thank God, He had brought me through two surgeries, chemo treatments, and radiation treatments.

During those winter months of driving to Radiation Treatment, God kept watch over me on those stormy and icy roads. He didn't allow me to have an accident. I am so happy He watched over me during that time.

One morning in particular, when I had to be on time for radiation treatments every day, the roads were so icy and dangerous that the roads leading to treatment had been closed down. I detoured onto another road and I was thanking God for watching over me, helping me to make it safely to my treatments.

During this period of time, I also lost my nephew and niece, Benjamin and Tamara Green in a bad car accident. This was a week before Christmas 2010. Going to radiation that morning and hearing it being talked about on the News was very devastating.

One of the nurses treating me that morning said that she had heard it on the News too. I couldn't hold back the tears. The nurses consoled me and I continued on with my treatment. God is so good; He will give you peace in the midst of the storm!

Chapter 14

What a Blessing!

A friend of ours once told my husband and me, "God can't use you until He breaks you." I found out that once He breaks you down a bit, then He blesses you. I can say during my breast cancer treatment, He poured down many blessings.

For one, He allowed me to retire early after 29 years of working for the State of Michigan/Department of Corrections. After chemotherapy and while getting ready for radiation, I received a notice in the mail from my employer. The letter noted that I qualified for "Early-Out Retirement," if I chose to. I couldn't believe it! I think I did a double take and read the letter over again.

After all those years of working, getting up early, going to bed late, driving in the rain, snow, ice, hail, and sleet in order to get to work, I now get this letter telling me I can retire and just rest. Oh, my God, what an awesome blessing! I only had to make up my mind as to what I wanted to do.

Of course, I consulted my husband and prayed about it sincerely. I think I was in a state of shock for a few days. Just to think, no more work, that sounded so good to me! All I needed to do was fill out all the required paperwork on the internet, send it in with the push of a button, and the process would begin.

As I sat and pondered over God's goodness, I would often think of those days working. Some days I just didn't want to be there. Every day at work would be the same routine day after day. However, the Lord knew my heart. Not that I didn't like work; not that I wasn't thankful to have a job. I was so grateful and so thankful to be working during that time. On the other hand, as I got older, my body was wearing down. I would get up tired. I didn't have as much energy as I once had. Then there's the younger workers waiting in the wings to take your desk and office. So God knew!

I had to come through breast cancer to get my blessing. Through all the tears, the pain, the disappointments, the fear, the not knowing what was going to happen to me, the crying, and the storms of life, I can say God brought me out!

I can truly say, when you are faced with a test, just go through it. There is a blessing on the other side.

Chapter 15

Symptoms

I had no symptoms to alert me I had breast cancer. I felt no lumps. I went to my mammogram appointment every year faithfully, and they found nothing. However, I missed going to my appointment in 2009. That year my Mom was sick fighting lung cancer and much of my time was about her, not me at that time. I did not follow up with my mammogram. However, like I stated earlier, a voice kept telling me to get checked. I kept putting it off until March of 2010. I know now that was the voice of God!

My Mom eventually passed away from complications of her cancer. She stayed in Hospice for a while where doctors had only given her a few months to live. Unknowingly after caring and seeing about my Mom, I would be diagnosed with cancer the following year. In life, sometimes, you just don't know!

The only thing that nagged me, was the pain in my right shoulder that would not subside. This is really what prompted me to go see my doctor, which in turned prompted me to request a mammogram authorization from my primary doctor. "God works in mysterious ways."

Even after getting the mammogram done, I felt fine. The nurse said she would contact me, if they found anything. Shortly thereafter, I did get that dreaded call, that they did see something, and wanted further x-rays and a biopsy. They said sometimes their findings could be wrong. I went to physical therapy and got a week's therapy for my shoulder pain, so that had been ruled out.

I went through the biopsy and x-rays, which was very scary and nerve wrecking because you just don't know what to expect. However, afterwards, I calmed down and felt fine. I felt everything would be alright! However, I was wrong!

Within a few days, I got that dreaded call at work. It was a Monday morning, and I was sitting at my desk. The voice stated, and I'll never forget, "Mrs. Wilson, I'm sorry you have cancer!"

Chapter 16

How Did I Cope?

First of all, I coped by trusting in my God! From the beginning when I was diagnosed, being scared and frightened, I told God, YOU take my hand as I follow where You lead me. During this coping process, God put songs in my spirit. Yes, I sat down during quiet times and wrote several songs of encouragement. Some of the songs God gave me are listed below:

On June 28, 2010 at 4:05 p.m., a song called "Road Untraveled."

> *"God says, Go, go take that road.*
> *Road untraveled is where I want you to go.*
>
> *I said, Lord, Oh Lord why me?*
> *The Lord said, Go, and I will give you the key.*
>
> *I said, Lord, keys to what?*
> *The Lord said, keys to my trust, keys to my love*
> *which comes from above.*
>
> *Keys to your sickness, which you don't understand.*
> *The keys to help you hold onto My hand.*
>
> *Keys to Life, which will set you free and*
> *will give you life more abundantly.*

Remember I am with you, I'm with you all the way.
Got your hand so tight you won't go astray.

I'm by your side over mountains and hills.
When danger comes, I just will
Speak, 'Peace be still.'

Road Untraveled is where I want you to go.
God says go, go take that road."

Another song God put in my spirit was earlier that same day, June 28, 2010, at 3:30 p.m., and is called "He Loves Me."

"I already knew He was great in my life.
I already knew my battles He would fight.

I already knew He was so sweet.
So, now I can say, He Loves Me.

(Chorus)
He loves me, Oh Yes, He loves me.
No matter how hard I fall,
He will be with me through it all.
He loves, Oh Yes, Jesus loves me.

I already knew He brightens up my days.
I already knew He makes ways out of no way.

I already knew He would see me through.
So, that's why I say, He loves me.

I already knew He heals the sick and raises the dead.
In His Word, 5,000 hungry souls he fed.

How Did I Cope?

He's the same God yesterday and today.
So, there's no doubt in my mind
He can and will make a way."

God put songs and hymns in my spirit to lift Him up in praise that in turn lifted my spirits up. The Scriptures in Psalm 22:3 say, that God dwells in the midst of praises. During the months and weeks feeling ill with my chemo treatments (nausea, dizziness, no appetite, weakness), God gave me songs of encouragement.

I would sit, oftentimes, on my back deck, notebook and pen in hand. I would just reminisce over God's goodness for hours and hours. I would think about all the prayers of my immediate family, church family, and friends. I would just write down about the goodness of God and His healing power.

There was one last song that God put in my spirit while sitting on my deck on July 4th, 2010. I began to look at nature: the green grass, blue sky, and hearing the little birds singing and flying around me. Also, the wind was blowing in my face, just a lovely afternoon! God spoke in my spirit and said, "WHY?"

Why do people worry so much?
Why are we so out of touch?

I look at nature and how it does its thing.
The grass grows green and the flowers do grow.
In the winter months, God allows it to snow.

The leaves are blowing just praising God in the wind.
They probably look at us people and I'm sure they grin.
Saying, why do people worry so much?

Why are we so out of touch?

If they only knew how close Jesus is.
If they only knew He's a breath away.
He comes to stay forever and always.
So, I ask you today WHY?"

I take comfort knowing God has my life under complete control. I walk in the way He leads me. I walk into my seasons of life, by faith in God; knowing assuredly I will survive! I'm walking with a winner, Jesus!

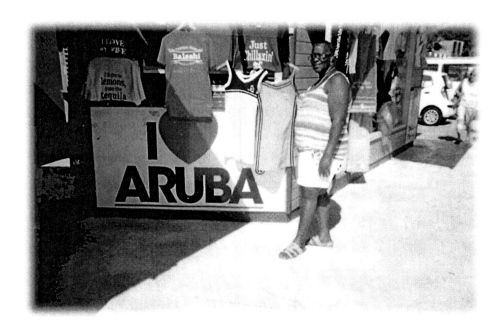

Chapter 17

I'm in Remission

As I write today, February 16, 2013, I have been in remission from breast cancer three years. I am retired from my State of Michigan job, for two years, after working for 29 years. Health-wise, I feel great! I have lost 40 pounds, not due to cancer sickness but because I needed to lose weight and stay healthy. I walk four times a week, and I try to eat right.

I have a passion for mentoring children, writing, singing, and traveling. Through the Grace of God, I have been able to do all of the above. Every now and then, I'll have an ache or pain. I was recently diagnosed with bone loss in my lower back. Tests revealed a blood clot in my ovary about a year ago. However, thank God that's been cleared up.

I try to stay busy. Two days a week, I tutor my seven-year-old nephew, Josh. Twice a month I make time for my Little Sister, Brionna (with Big Brothers, Big Sisters). I have a little god child, Justyce, who is 8 months old that I visit twice a week. I sing in my church choir, Excellent Praise, second Sunday of every month. I love when my husband and I get to travel to places like Myrtle Beach, Las Vegas, Florida, Mexico, Dominican Republic and many more places. I try to make time with my three adult children, Dionne (son-in-law Kirk) Walter, and Daniel. Note: Since starting this book, I have a grandson (Corey) 9 months old, who I love so much! Corey was born November 6, 2014.

I'm living my life to the fullest. I'm putting God first in my life and giving Him praise each and every day. I love life! I love living! I love God!

Chapter 18

Dedicated to My Sister, the Late Linda Kay Hall

My younger sister, Linda Kay Hall, passed away on June 11, 2015, Thursday at 4:20 p.m. She was only 53 years old, a wife, mother, sister, RN, student and well-loved by many. She died from complications of Leukemia (cancer of the blood).

She was diagnosed in October of 2014. She began experiencing breathing problems and bruises appeared on her body which eventually got worse. She decided to go to Emergency one Sunday afternoon after Church. Immediately, after some tests were done she needed a blood transfusion, x-rays were done, and without a doubt, she was admitted that day.

Reports we received from her husband, Percy, was that her condition was very serious. Although at that time, the family did not know it was Leukemia. We, as a family, started to pray! Within a week, we learned what her condition was. She had to undergo chemo therapy along with the blood transfusions, and a spinal tap. The spinal tap was very painful; Linda would later tell us.

The chemo caused her to lose her hair. She became very weak, lost her appetite, and had the usual side effects that chemo causes.

At the last, she needed a bone marrow transplant. This required a donor which had to be a family member. The blood type had to be a complete match with Linda's (O Positive). Thank God our youngest brother, Anthony, the last out of 12 children, was the perfect match! The bone marrow transplant went fine. Linda was recovering fairly well, and we all were so hopeful.

However, within about a week, the bone marrow process left her body very weak. She began to get rashes on her body, sores on her tongue, she couldn't eat like she wanted. On top of all the above, her immune system was very low. She became susceptible to various infections.

We had to wear masks and hospital gowns whenever we went to see her. We had to wash our hands making sure we had no colds or flu. If you came in coughing or sneezing, you were not allowed to see her.

Linda did, however, contract at least two infections and was transferred to ICU on both occasions. The first was a skin infection on her leg which required surgery. She was in ICU for about a week. The second was meningitis in her brain. This required her to be put on a ventilator, feeding tube, and a breathing tube. She was unconscious for several days, not responding to commands. However, eventually after about a week, she started to squeeze hands and nod her head when asked to do something.

About a month or two after this, Linda began to get a little better. She was able to come home. I got the chance to visit her on her birthday, March 22, 2015, on a Sunday after Church.

Dedicated to My Sister, the Late Linda Kay Hall

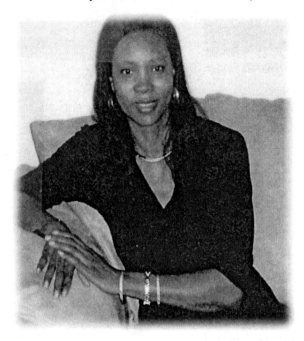

She was at home recuperating from her first bone marrow transplant (eventually she had to have a second bone marrow transplant). We talked for two hours about her illness, how she was determined, with God's help, to fight it out! She was so happy the rash from the transplant was clearing up on her face and arms, and the sores in her mouth were gone.

She was happy to be home from the hospital. She had been in the hospital during Christmas, New Year's, and she was happy they finally let her come home, just in time for her 53rd birthday. My husband and I asked her what she wanted us to bring her to eat; she requested KFC, a Squirt Pop; and of course, we got her a Birthday Card.

As we ended our two-hour conversation with Linda, she told us, "I want to live!" She said she was doing everything within her power to stay healthy, taking her medications, making her doctor's appointments, trying to eat right, and she was, as well as we, were hopeful things were looking better on her behalf.

However, within a week, Linda had to return to the hospital. After one of her doctor's appointments her blood count was low and she was admitted to start treatments over again. Linda eventually stopped eating, and even communicating to her husband, family, nurses, doctors and everyone. She slept all day. She would occasionally nod her head, yes or no. When she communicated, it would only be a whisper. She would occasionally open her eyes. I perceived that she was ready to go to that better place!

I remember her words, "I want to live." Naturally, I know she's not with us, but spiritually, she is living, alive, and well with Jesus. I realize and know, that to everything there really is a season. I'm so glad I got the chance to spend 53 years with my sister, Linda. I loved you Dear Sister, but God loved you Best! Rest in Peace!

Chapter 19

Life Lessons

Lesson 1: Put your faith in God!

As I went through this season of sickness, many days I had to truly trust in God's Word to bring me through. On the days I didn't feel like getting out of bed, I could hear the voice of God saying, "Just get up and start moving." I'm glad I had my faith to lean on when I received that diagnosis. If you don't know Him, just ask. He is right there beside you. Believe it!

Lesson 2: Appreciate your family and friends

I learned that family is so important. They were my support system. My husband and daughter were there for both my surgeries and my chemo treatments. My Pastor and Church family sent up prayers on my behalf. My co-workers were there for that shoulder to cry on when I first received my diagnosis at work. I'll always appreciate the surprise birthday party my brothers and sisters threw me to help keep my spirits up! Don't take those who love you for granted.

Lesson 3: Get your mammograms!

Because my mother was in hospice suffering from lung cancer, I missed my mammogram in 2009. I know life can get busy, but don't procrastinate! GET CHECKED!

Lesson 4: Encourage others

Be ready to give your testimony to encourage and inspire others. When a friend of mine was battling cancer I encouraged her to "Keep moving. Get up, get dressed, and put your makeup on. Go buy some pretty scarves, or a wig, get a new outfit. Just keep living!" She later told me that she needed to hear that and it helped her to make a turn around that day. Be ready to share how God brought you through.

Lesson 5: Stay positive

There is always hope! See yourself getting better. See yourself as a survivor. Claim life! Talk life! Be around others who have overcome cancer. I loved seeing women who have been in remission from breast cancer for five or ten years. They gave me hope that I could get there too!

My Season, My Thoughts

Well, as I conclude this book writing portion of this season by sharing my experiences from my breast cancer journey, I can truly say there have been good and bad times. I would describe it as interesting, amazing, awesome, some good days, some bad days, some ups, some downs, and some painful and some disappointing moments.

To quote Andre Crouch,[3] "Through it all, I've learned to trust in Jesus. I've learned to trust in God." Truly God has brought me through, thus far. I am a Survivor! I am claiming victory each and every day.

I continue my annual mammograms, oncology checkups, bone density checkups, port flushes, and CT Scans. In claiming victory, there are annual checkups I have to abide by.

As long as I have breath and life in this body, I will keep praising God! He brought me through this season in my life for a reason. At the end of the day, it's not about ME! It's about being a testimony for someone else who will be diagnosed with breast cancer or any other cancer. The big picture is bigger than, "little old me." It's about helping others overcome and learning to cope while battling cancer.

I hope this book does just that. I hope it encourages someone. I hope it uplifts and enlightens someone to keep moving through it all. I hope it gives others the strength to always remember God

All of us will have our seasons of difficulty through life. In the Old Testament, the book of Ecclesiastes, Chapter 3:1-11 says:

*"To everything there is a season,
and a time to every purpose under the sun.*

---

[3] Andre Crouch. *Through it All* Billy Graham Crusade, in New Mexico, 1975

A time to be born, and a time to die;

A time to plant, and a time to pluck up that which is planted;

A time to kill, and a time to heal;

A time to breakdown, and a time to build up;

A time to weep, and a time to laugh;

A time to mourn, and a time to dance;

A time to cast a way stones,

and a time to gather stones together;

A time to embrace, and a time to refrain from embracing;

A time to get, and a time to lose;

A time to keep, and a time to case away;

A time to rend, and a time to sew;

A time to keep silence, and a time to speak;

A time to love, and a time to hate;

A time of war, and a time of peace;

He hath made everything beautiful in its time."

May this Scripture inspire you as it did me. It spoke to my spirit as I went through this season of life, overcoming breast cancer. I made it with God's help, and you can too! Be forever blessed!

Author Bio

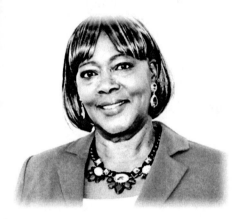

Margin Wilson is making her writing debut as she shares her victory over breast cancer. Raised in a family with twelve siblings, Margin was surrounded by teaching from God's Word. Sunday morning worship, Monday night prayer, Wednesday night bible study, Thursday Junior Missionary Service and youth choir rehearsals kept faith in God in the forefront. In fact, church would be where she met the love of her life.

Educated in Detroit Public Schools with an Associate Degree in Business, Margin worked inside the prison system for the Department of Corrections for 29 years.

Recent years have found Margin's focus on ministry and mentoring. In addition to her love of writing and singing, she enjoys traveling around the world!

She says that being diagnosed with breast cancer in 2010 has inspired her to minister and share her story with others. With a new zest for life, Margin says that the season of sickness she endured has made her even stronger!

Married for 36 years, Margin and her husband, Walter, live in southeast Michigan and are the parents of three adult children and one grandson.

To contact Mrs. Wilson for speaking engagements:

Mrs. Margin Wilson
c/o PriorityONE Publications
P.O. Box 34722 • Detroit, MI 48224 USA
www.MarginWilson.com
734-707-3636

CPSIA information can be obtained
at www.ICGtesting.com
Printed in the USA
FFOW02n0712190218
45156247-45652FF

9 781933 972541

It's NOT the End of the World!
Life Lessons of a Breast Cancer Survivor

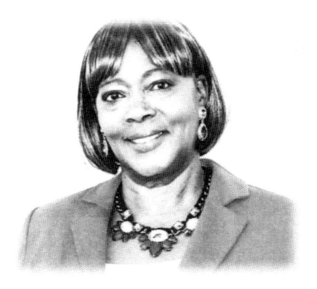

By Margin Wilson

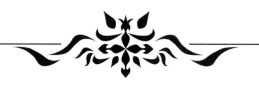

Life Lessons

Lesson 1: Put your faith in God!

As I went through this season of sickness, many days I had to truly trust in God's Word to bring me through. On the days I didn't feel like getting out of bed, I could hear the voice of God saying, "Just get up and start moving." I'm glad I had my faith to lean on when I received that diagnosis. If you don't know Him, just ask. He is right there beside you. Believe it!

Lesson 2: Appreciate your family and friends

I learned that family is so important. They were my support system. My husband and daughter were there for both my surgeries and my chemo treatments. My Pastor and Church family sent up prayers on my behalf. My co-workers were there for that shoulder to cry on when I first received my diagnosis at work. I'll always appreciate the surprise birthday party my brothers and sisters threw me to help keep my spirits up! Don't take those who love you for granted.

Lesson 3: Get your mammograms!

Because my mother was in hospice suffering from lung cancer, I missed my mammogram in 2009. I know life can get busy, but don't procrastinate! **GET CHECKED!**

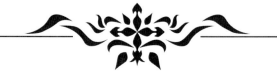

Lesson 4: Encourage others

Be ready to give your testimony to encourage and inspire others. When a friend of mine was battling cancer I encouraged her to "Keep moving. Get up, get dressed, and put your makeup on. Go buy some pretty scarves, or a wig, get a new outfit. Just keep living!" She later told me that she needed to hear that and it helped her to make a turn around that day. Be ready to share how God brought you through.

Lesson 5: Stay positive

There is always hope! See yourself getting better. See yourself as a survivor. Claim life! Talk life! Be around others who have overcome cancer. I loved seeing women who have been in remission from breast cancer for five or ten years. They gave me hope that I could get there too!

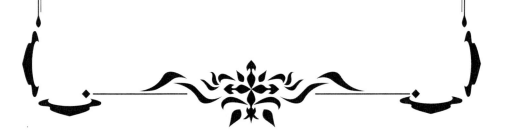

Author Bio

Margin Wilson is making her writing debut as she shares her victory over breast cancer. Raised in a family with twelve siblings, Margin was surrounded by teaching from God's Word.

Sunday morning worship, Monday night prayer, Wednesday night bible study, Thursday Junior Missionary Service and youth choir rehearsals kept faith in God in the forefront. In fact, church would be where she met the love of her life.

Educated in Detroit Public Schools with an Associate Degree in Business, Margin worked inside the prison system for the Department of Corrections for 29 years.

Recent years have found Margin's focus on ministry and mentoring. In addition to her love of writing and singing, she enjoys traveling around the world!

She says that being diagnosed with breast cancer in 2010 has inspired her to minister and share her story with others. With a new zest for life, Margin says that the season of sickness she endured has made her even stronger!

Married for 36 years, Margin and her husband, Walter, live in southeast Michigan and are the parents of three adult children and one grandson.